A JOURNEY THROUGH CANCER

By
MELANIE BONE, M.D.
RICHARD M. CROMIE, D.D., Ph.D.

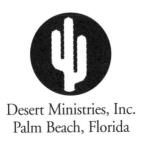

Desert Ministries, Inc.
Palm Beach, Florida

A Journey Through Cancer

First Edition
©Copyright 2002 by
Desert Ministries, Inc.
P.O. Box 788
Palm Beach, FL 33480
ISBN 0-914733-29-X

Printed by Eagle Graphic Services, Fort Lauderdale, Florida

⁓ℓ. PREFACE .℘⁓

For nearly a score of years, Desert Ministries Inc., the publisher of this expanding series of books for people in times of special need, has offered a well used booklet titled _How To Live With Cancer_. For its time it was acceptable. We were often told that it was helpful for those who had been diagnosed with cancer, as well as to their friends and family. We revised it three times. I was the author. I have been a pastor for forty two years, frequently ministering to cancer patients, their families and friends, and to Doctors, nurses, and health care professionals. The booklet served its purpose.

But, in recent years, I kept remembering two comments from friends, separated in time by over twenty years, which prompted me to publish a new book. When I moved to Florida in the summer of 1983, I met a man there, Byrd Booth, an active member of the committee which invited Peggy and me to move to Ft. Lauderdale from Pittsburgh. Sadly at that time he had been diagnosed with a severe cancer of the brain which took his life within the next few months. Byrd's death saddened us tremendously. He was quite complimentary prior to that on my then new booklet on cancer. But after his genuinely nice words, he added "It is obvious however, that it was written by one who does not have the disease." I was not sure what he meant. But, I heard his words and remembered.

Then move all the way up to 2001. I sent a copy of the revised booklet to an old Pittsburgh friend who had experienced a recent struggle with cancer. She responded immediately, almost indignantly, "I don't need to know how to <u>live</u> with cancer. My cancer is gone. I am a survivor!" Halleluiah. Amen.

That did it! Twenty years have brought significant changes in cancer treatment, as well as in attitudes toward the disease. I decided that DMI needed help in offering a new book on cancer. In the time and providence of God, it was then that I met Dr. Melanie Bone. Melanie and her husband, Bill who is a member of the DMI Board, are good friends. Melanie not only has great skills in communication, but she is a widely revered gynecologist and obstetrician who has treated, and I will add "ministered to," endless numbers of women with cancer. She also (to satisfy my Pittsburgh friend) is a "Cancer Survivor." Melanie has gone through "*The Journey.*" God bless her. She is an inspiration to me and countless others.

We at Desert Ministries are grateful to all of those who care about our work. Especially in the publication of this volume, we thank two donors, one a Foundation, one an individual person who prefers to be anonymous. They provided significant contributions to fund the printing of this book. A list of other books available is printed at the end of this publication.

I know you will enjoy and be richly touched by _A Journey Through Cancer_. I cannot read it without tears of joy forming in my eyes. We send you our love and prayers. Meanwhile, God bless you and keep you in His care.

Reverend Richard M. Cromie, Ph.D., D.D
President, Desert Ministries, Inc.

TABLE OF CONTENTS

PART 1
A PERSONAL JOURNEY
MELANIE BONE, M.D.

PART 2
SIX LESSONS FOR LIVING WITH CANCER
RICHARD M. CROMIE, D.D.

ABOUT THE AUTHORS

PART 1

A
PERSONAL
JOURNEY

Introduction

When Dr. Cromie approached me about re-writing his book, _How to Live with Cancer_, the project appealed to me for several reasons. I am a practicing obstetrician/gynecologist and a breast cancer survivor. I was also an English literature major at Georgetown University, and I thought it would be a good use of my education to try to write something longer than my usual column for _Vive_, a regional women's magazine. In his typical congenial way, Dr. Cromie gave me _carte blanche_ to work on my own. I jotted down a few ideas and promptly let the project simmer for a few months.

In April 2002, I took a trip to Phoenix, Arizona, with some girlfriends. I had been to Scottsdale before and remembered there was a short but strenuous hike up Squaw Peak just a few minutes away from our hotel. I awakened early one morning, put on my running shoes and went off to find the trailhead. Picking my way up the well-worn, rocky trail, I started thinking about the book. I couldn't help but wonder how many other hikers had been touched by cancer.

When I reached the summit, I plopped down and

enjoyed the beautiful panoramic views. A young man came up and sat down next to me. Our conversation started with the natural beauty of Arizona and ended up about his father-in-law's renal cell cancer. Diagnosed 8 years earlier, the man was still being treated for cancer, but maintained a positive outlook and a good quality of life. When I mentioned that I was a cancer survivor too, the young hiker was surprised: he thought I looked too young to have had cancer.

On the walk back down the steep trail, I felt a little sorry for myself. Yes, I was too young for cancer, and had four children under the age of 7 to raise. As I tried to work through some of my negative feelings, I took note of the other hikers. Some were all business, never looking at anything but their own feet. Some stopped and took in the vistas at the various rest points. Others actually jogged to the summit and immediately turned around and zipped back down. The similarity between jogging and cancer struck me, since we cancer patients face the "hike of a lifetime" when we deal with our illness. The number of steps, the speed, and the route differ from patient to patient, but our ultimate destination is the same: survival. How we are changed during the trek depends on the road we take.

The analogy of cancer as a trek or a journey has been used before with good reason. It is a journey that in some ways parallels the journey of life. Prior to diagnosis, we are like innocent children. At the moment of diagnosis, we lose that innocence. We then become educated about cancer before going through a period of difficult decisions about treatment options. This is much like adolescence. During treatment we become accustomed to the idea of

4

our disease as a part of our lives and deal with it as adults. For most cancer patients, the end of treatment is similar to retirement—eagerly anticipated as well as dreaded. Survivorship is like the twilight years—fulfilling, yet marked by anxiety. Recurrence or terminal illness brings on the need to discuss end-of-life issues, which all of us will face some day.

Although part of this book is a retelling of my personal story, I have used myself as a jumping off point to help patients and their families in their own struggle with cancer. I hope this small book is helpful in the journey.

M Bone

Melanie Bone, M.D.

$\sim\!\!\approx$ 1 $\approx\!\!\sim$

LIFE BEFORE CANCER

I include a chapter about life before a cancer diagnosis only as a reference. I remember the day I was diagnosed. Suddenly, my entire life before cancer ceased to exist. The irony is that I was the SAME person on the day AFTER diagnosis that I was on the day BEFORE diagnosis, except that on the day after diagnosis I was aware there was cancer in my body. I recall thinking that, "ignorance is bliss," was very apropos. I felt robbed of my innocence. "Cancer is a disease of old people with old cells. I have a 2-year old son. I am too young for cancer," I thought. I was shattered. My mortality stared me in the face.

Most of us live without confronting our own mortality until much later in life. Unless you have been exposed to such a trauma, it is hard to comprehend how it feels to understand that life as you know it is gone forever. There is little that compares with the horror of hearing the words, "You have cancer."

It may be nearly impossible to remember your life before cancer for a long, long time. Eventually, though, life returns to a new normality, and most of us go back to our old ways. Life after cancer often turns out to be the same life as before cancer. With a little good luck and a lot of good medicine, the goal is to have a more difficult time remembering your life during cancer than your life before or after it.

~ 2 ~

COMING TO DIAGNOSIS

The time between normal life, when cancer is suspected but not proven, and the day of diagnosis needs to be mentioned because it is full of mixed emotions and can be highly stressful for patients and their families. It can last a few minutes, days, weeks, or even months. During this time, patients have so many tumultuous thoughts and feelings that their behavior often changes, and their loved ones may misinterpret what is happening.

Fear, of course, tops the list of emotions. I believe that many cancer patients somehow know that a terrible problem exists before it is diagnosed. My mind played games to protect me from this realization. I remember thinking that I looked thin and drawn in the months before my diagnosis, but I attributed it to the stress of a new job and four little children at home. When I began to see skin changes on my breast and suspected they were from cancer, I was frozen with fear. To this day I am not sure how I made the decision to have a biopsy, but I am certain that my premonitions delayed my diagnosis.

Along with my fear and suspicion, I told myself not to be an alarmist. My family used to tease me about how I exaggerate everything, so I could not help but think that maybe I was overreacting. After all, I was able to work long hours, run five miles and take care of my family, so I could not be very sick. I kept telling myself that the swollen gland *(in my left armpit)* was probably from a virus or a shaving nick.

At some point, however, most cancer patients find that their suspicions and fears outweigh their mind's attempt to maintain normalcy. Then a diagnosis is made.

There are some patients for whom a cancer diagnosis comes as a total surprise, but in my years as a physician, I have met very few. Some suffer terrible guilt, as if they were out of tune with their body, or would have suspected something earlier. I tell them that even people who suspect they have cancer often procrastinate. Most of the time, it has little impact on treatment or survival.

3

THE DAY OF DIAGNOSIS

No matter what road we take, there is no question that the day of diagnosis is excruciating. Personally, I was very happy to be under the influence of anesthesia drugs when my doctor came in to tell me. She didn't use the word cancer. "It isn't good," she said, and began to sob.

Giving this news is almost as difficult as receiving it, and doctors have a hard time mentioning the word "cancer." How doctors deliver the news varies. We have not perfected the art of giving a cancer diagnosis.

Being on the receiving end of the cancer news is like getting hit by lightening. At first, the word "cancer" causes shock. In me, it produced a visceral reaction with nausea, dizziness, sweating and palpitations. Most cancer patients have a similar experience. The first thought that crosses your mind is that you are going to die. This fear and the physical symptoms that accompany it can last for a long time. As a physician and a survivor, I am in favor of using anti-anxiety medications to alleviate these feelings of dread. They are not a long-term solution, but they can be invaluable in the short run.

Side-by-side with fear comes a sense of disbelief. Many patients feel they are in a dream. This is a classic example of the coping skill called denial, and it gives the brain time to digest the news and confront it while the reality of the situation soaks in.

Sometimes our loved ones and friends make comments that cause hurt and anger. One friend told me she thought I had been looking "gaunt" for a while. Although I knew she meant well, I wondered why hadn't she said something that might have brought me to diagnosis sooner? Such friends are really well meaning and have no idea that their words produce feelings of guilt about our own tendency to ignore important symptoms.

In the days immediately following diagnosis, most patients cannot bring themselves to talk openly about their disease. They try to keep it a secret, as if ignoring it might make it go away. The diagnosis is simply too raw to face. Over time, they generally muster the internal strength needed to dominate their fear. Most patients eventually develop a relationship with their disease that permits them to speak openly or even joke about it. But this does not happen overnight.

4

AFTER DIAGNOSIS

The days after diagnosis are a whirlwind of activity. Doctors appointments, staging tests and information gathering provide a much-needed distraction. As this process unfolds, the brain assimilates the diagnosis and becomes accustomed to it.

For cancer patients who are unfamiliar with medicine, the days can be fraught with confusion and anxiety. Not only are you faced with having a deadly disease, but you must also decide how best to treat it. Most physicians present their patients with a treatment plan or several treatment options. But the patient may also be deluged with other opinions, some asked for and some not. Many turn to the Internet for information. The result is mass confusion. I chose the opinion of the doctors I respected most and never looked back.

There is a tendency among cancer patients to want the BEST care, even if it means traveling to a "mecca" of cancer care. While this approach is definitely advisable for rare forms of cancer, it is not necessarily the best course of action for more common forms. Being treated in your own community has many advantages. I recommend going to a nearby cancer center or an oncologist who has access to treatment protocols from a cancer center. I did, because I felt totally confident that I would receive the same medications, and I would have the added benefit of being near my friends and family. Their support more than made up for any possible difference in medical care.

Part of the post-diagnosis activity is the metastatic work-up. This usually includes scans and tests to determine whether or not the cancer has spread from its site of origin. These tests are bittersweet: negative tests make you feel like you have avoided the guillotine, but lying on the table awaiting the results is torture. I needed anti-anxiety medicine to keep from jumping out of my skin.

Once all tests are done, it is time to sit down with your physician or a team of physicians to choose a course of treatment. This may be the best time to bring another set of ears into the discussion. I was interested in having the most aggressive treatment possible, so the only decision I really had to make was to choose the hospital for my surgery. The date was dependent on the surgeons' availability. By relinquishing control of the situation to experts in whom I had complete faith, I was free to concentrate on dealing with other matters.

For some patients, the decision whether or not to share the news about their disease with people outside their immediate family causes a great deal of anxiety. I was compelled to tell my patients the truth. I had hired a new doctor to join my practice, she was scheduled to start a month later, but agreed to start earlier to help me out. Without hesitation she jumped in – seeing my full schedule of patients and performing my surgeries. For this I am eternally grateful. Some patients chose to go to a different practice. Most either saw my new partner or came back when I did. Honesty about a cancer diagnosis was the right approach for me, but every person is different For example, I have two friends who are doctors. When they were treated for cancer they did not inform their colleagues or their patients until after they returned to work.

After the treatment plan is determined, there is usually a short period of time before the treatment actually begins. It is wise to make good use of this time. Although I was anxious to get the cancer out of my body, I found I was incredibly busy making preparations for my business and planning for recovery from bilateral mastectomies. The last few days did feel like an eternity. I actually got excited the day before surgery, much like people do before a big celebration. I even had a manicure, pedicure and facial—a gift from coworkers (and a good one, I might add). I told myself that my surgery would be the first day of the rest of my new life.

5

GETTING TREATMENT

Surgery, chemotherapy and radiation are the most common treatments for cancer. As a surgeon, I was taught that, "a chance to cut is a chance to cure." Not all patients agree, and many are terrified of surgery. I was happy to have a cancer amenable to surgical removal. Sure, there was postoperative pain and some rough times, but for the most part, I was able to grin and bear it. Setting goals helped a lot. For example, there was a party for the parents of incoming kindergartners at my daughter's new school only two weeks after my surgery. I promised myself that I would be there, and I was! It is easy to fall into a "woe-is-me" attitude after cancer surgery, but it does no good. It certainly will not improve the rate at which you get better, and it can impair your immune system, which is essential in fighting any cancer cells that remain behind.

Unlike surgery, chemotherapy really scared me. I couldn't help but remember my experience with it during my internship. Right out of medical school and green behind the ears, I was assigned to the oncology ward. I remember a young breast cancer patient who had been admitted for her second round of chemotherapy. She was in a wheelchair coming down the hall to be admitted and vomiting copiously into an emesis basin in anticipation of her upcoming treatment. Although the pretreatment drugs used today virtually eliminate that degree of nausea and vomiting, I still dreaded having chemotherapy.

When I arrived for the first of eight treatments (every 21 days for approximately six months), I was shivering uncontrollably. Luckily, the infusion nurses were incredibly skilled at alleviating fear and slipped some anti-anxiety medicine in my port (an internal IV in my chest) that left me smiling and placid for the remainder of the day.

After I was finished with my first chemo session, it was strange to leave and not really feel much different. My husband and I went to lunch, and then I went home to wait for the onslaught. Much to my surprise, the chemotherapy itself did not cause any immediate side effects. The drugs I took to avoid the side effects, however, caused mood swings, stomach upset and insomnia.

It took a little time for the chemotherapy to catch up with me. After three or four treatments, I felt extremely fatigued. I would pretreat myself with steroids at home to lessen the nausea, and this made me feel "wired." One morning, I cleaned my closets at 2 a.m. I could not taste much because the chemo destroyed my tastebuds, but I craved chocolate nonetheless. How disappointing to pop a Hershey's kiss in my mouth and not taste it! When the steroids wore off, my period of hyperactivity would end, and acute depression would set in.

Most cancers have a pre-determined treatment schedule. Patients can check off the number of remaining treatments. I was supposed to finish my chemotherapy in January, just in time to participate in the Race for the Cure, a breast cancer event. During my first few chemotherapy treatments, my blood counts held strong, and I got excited about the race.

Unfortunately, a chemotherapy schedule can be delayed by abnormal blood counts or infections. Such delays can produce intense emotions. I never imagined how bad I would feel when I had my first disappointing counts. My oncologist canceled my treatment, and I realized I would not finish my chemotherapy in time for the race. I felt like a failure and cried hysterically in the infusion room.

When a cancer patient's white blood cell count plummets, they are at risk for a life-threatening infection, even if they feel fine. The oncologists may start antibiotics and forbid eating fresh fruits and vegetables. I also was told to stay away from my young children, who might carry a virus. I had to move out of my house and into a friend's house more than once because of this. The first time scared me, but after that I told myself that it was like going on a vacation. In fact, I let my friend dote on me, and it felt wonderful!

The best advice I can give someone on chemotherapy is to try to stay upbeat and flexible. I was not finished with my chemotherapy by the Race for the Cure, but I participated. I managed to find a wheelchair, and my nurse pushed me when I was unable to walk.

Radiation therapy was a piece of cake compared with chemotherapy. The doctors told me I would feel tired, but it was much less exhausting than I expected. Yes, there were some skin changes to treat, but slathering myself with special lotions three times a day was easy to do. The hardest part was arriving at the radiation center on time for 33 days in a row. I really enjoyed meeting the other patients, and we developed a kind of camaraderie. When one of us did not show up, we became concerned. When someone's treatments ended, we toasted the event with coffee in the waiting area. It was a very special kind of support.

I could hardly believe it when my radiation treatments were over. I was about to enter the world of survivorship.

6

THE QUESTION OF ALTERNATIVE THERAPY

Alternative treatments for cancer have been available for a long time. Some are useful, and some are not. Many patients feel that their doctors will not approve of alternative treatments, so they hide them from their doctors or eschew traditional medicine in favor of them. In reality, most physicians feel that some alternative treatments complement traditional medicine; hence a new area of medicine called CAM (Complementary and Alternative Medicine) has been developed.

The danger of using alternative remedies without telling your oncologist is that they can interfere with chemotherapy or radiation therapy. For example, most radiation oncologists ask their patients not to use antioxidant vitamins while they are undergoing radiation treatments. The reason is that antioxidants protect the cancer cells from the effects of the radiation. Once the cancer cells have been killed off, most doctors would agree that resuming antioxidants supplements would help strengthen the remaining healthy cells.

Some herbal remedies have been shown to be effective in cancer treatments, but so have traditional therapies. The difference is that few scientific studies have been conducted comparing herbal or other alternative treatments with conventional ones. Therefore, there is no proof that these treatments are as good as or better than chemotherapy, surgery or radiation. Until such studies are done, it is premature to suggest that cancer patients should decline traditional methods in favor of an alternative route. If you are inclined to try non-traditional treatments first, I suggest you weigh the consequences carefully. Remember that patients who elect less aggressive or alternative first-line therapies and suffer a recurrence often experience tremendous guilt and regret.

Lest you feel that I may be against alternative medicines, let me tell you that I take *uña de gato* (Cat's Claw, an Amazon rainforest herb that is an immune enhancer), grapeseed extract and pine bark extract (powerful antioxidants) and zinc supplements. I believe these are not likely to hurt me and may well help me. I have read extensively about other therapies, and know I could spend a lot of time and money on other options. At this point, however, I will choose to wait for more studies to be done.

Non-medical complementary therapies also deserve mention. Massage, therapeutic touch, and craniosacral therapy can all be beneficial in the right setting. Other forms of immune modulation, such as music therapy or art therapy, can also be helpful as well as soothing. I often engaged in visualization exercises, listened to affirmation tapes and meditated to stimulate my own "natural killer" cells to attack any residual cancer. There are many of these therapies that help the mind to overcome both physical and emotional challenges of treatment.

7

SURVIVORSHIP

There are many mixed emotions about finishing cancer treatment. There is joy and happiness for making it through. There is also physical, emotional and psychological exhaustion. Moreover, there is fear that cancer might return. While the overwhelming feeling is that the worst is over, you are suddenly faced with trying to reestablish normalcy. This can be very hard.

I felt a huge sense of accomplishment to have survived the treatment. My colleague and office staff threw an end-of-treatment party complete with cake and good cheer. My children were excited that I no longer needed to run off to the "radiation rocketship" every day and would be able to see more of them. I felt everyone else's joy for me. That is why I could not tell them about the dark feeling I had inside. The rituals of treatments were comforting and served as a lifeline. So long as I was taking poisons to kill the cancer, I felt safe. Now there was a chance it would come back. I immediately realized how bittersweet it is to be a survivor.

Each patient deals with survivorship differently. For

me, the urge to become a cancer activist was overwhelming. I knew I would feel better if I could prevent even one young mother from getting breast cancer. I quickly joined charitable breast cancer organizations and used my position as a physician-survivor to help. Although I often felt worn out, I pushed myself to attend meetings, write letters to politicians, solicit donations, and join charitable Boards. I admit that I was a little manic. Today, I know this behavior is fairly common and takes over many patients' lives, much to the dismay of their spouses and children. Instead of taking Disney vacations, the whole family gets dragged to walks, runs, marches, and other cancer advocacy functions.

Many families who have been disrupted by cancer treatments view the end of treatment as a chance to normalize. They are thrilled that routines will return to the way they were, and that cancer can finally take a back seat to other life events. The problem is that for most survivors, cancer can never take a back seat—at least, not for a long time. It is a companion forever. This difference in perception can be problematic. At one point, my husband began to wonder if there was ever going to be life AFTER breast cancer. I told him that it would always impact our lives, and the best I could offer was the hope that if I survived long enough, the impact might diminish over time.

It is impossible not to look in the mirror every day and wonder if a few cancer cells are still lurking somewhere. Every backache, headache or physical ailment causes fear of recurrence. As a physician, I see many long-term survivors. They tell me their fear lessens over time but never disappears. There is little you can do about it, except to try using medication, faith or distraction to control it. Other survivors understand what it feels like, and that is why support groups are so successful.

Finding an outlet for feelings of anxiety is an important part of survivorship. The outlet may take the form of advocacy and volunteering, particularly in early survivorship. Sometimes, however, it expresses itself in an intense need to live life to the fullest. This can mean taking on too many things at once. When that happens, burnout is almost guaranteed. In my second year as a survivor, I met a woman who had started a cancer survivors' newsletter. She was a member of many volunteer organizations, and was always the one to organize events and serve on the Board. Eventually, she couldn't sustain it and gave it all up to devote more time to her family. Even worse is when the stress of survivorship can lead to drug or alcohol abuse. Families and friends of survivors should watch out for this type of behavior so they can intervene early if the need arises.

8

DEALING WITH RECURRENCE

While all cancer survivors suffer from fear of recurrence, most are ready to put up a good fight if it happens. The will to live is generally so strong that it far outweighs the fear of treatment-related suffering. I have talked to many repeat survivors who say that the difference between the first time and recurrence is that the fear of the unknown is gone.

In many ways, treatment for a recurrence is less agonizing. For one, the recurrence is often localized and can be treated surgically. Also, second-line chemotherapy drugs may be less aggressive than first-line drugs and are, therefore, better tolerated.

Setting short-term goals in the face of a recurrence may be wise. It is better to focus on achieving another remission than worrying about being cured. This makes sense, given the rapid changes in new cancer treatments. Only a few years ago, Gleevic did not exist, and today the drug can put some terminally ill cancer patients in remission. Such scientific advances keep us hopeful. I still remember a neighbor, an oncologist whose own son was struggling with leukemia, telling me that if I could get five years of remission from my first round of treatment, a whole new set of drugs would be available to treat a recurrence.

Of course, there is an unspoken fear of death when cancer recurs a recurrence occurs. Thoughts that the cancer might not be controllable and might ultimately be fatal creep in and out. We hear about how important it is to think positively. A positive attitude has been shown to boost the immune system, and there is no doubt that the immune system has a profound impact on cancer. Many patients practice visualization exercises and recite affirmations, both of which are thought to stimulate the immune system. The immune mechanism involves "natural killer cells" in our bloodstream which seek out the cancer cells and destroy them. Scientists are now designing therapies to increase the power of these killer cells using antibodies to specific markers on the cancer cells (antigens). These drugs can target the cancer cells exclusively.

It is not surprising that many patients become depressed during a recurrence. This is a natural reaction. Sometimes it may be related to the initial choice of treatments. When patients elect to have less-intensive therapy the first time around and suffer a recurrence, it may be accompanied by a sense of guilt. One reason I chose aggressive treatment was to avoid feeling guilty, should I have a recurrence. Every day, I look in the mirror and tell myself that if my cancer returns, there was nothing more I could have done to stop it. If I were faced with the decision again, I would take the same course. I realize that not all patients feel the way I do, but guilt serves no purpose, and dealing with recurrence is hard enough without it.

9

END-OF-LIFE ISSUES

End-of-life issues are hard for me to discuss. No one has a crystal ball to know when he or she will die. When cancer is not treatable or progresses despite treatment, it is time to stop therapy and take another approach. This is one of the most challenging times for physicians. On one hand, they do not want to be prematurely gloomy; on the other hand, they do not want to prolong useless suffering.

I have had many conversations with my oncologist about this dilemma. No doctor wants to take away hope, but many fear that telling patients their cancer is terminal may perpetuate a self-fulfilling prophecy and hasten the patient's death. This thought process may be an unconscious driving force behind the tendency for doctors to avoid predicting how much time a patient has left. In defense of the oncologists I know, I would have to say that they try very hard not to sidestep end-of-life discussions, but by training they are more apt to continue life-prolonging therapies than not.

Having said this, it is not always clear to doctors how long a patient will survive after treatments are halted. A book entitled, "Remarkable Recovery," gives many examples of patients whose doctors gave up on them, and who were still alive 20 years later. However, clinical experience goes a long way in helping identify patients who are likely to succumb to cancer.

Many practical things can be done that make it easier for everyone involved in the care of a terminally ill patient. Since the patient's wishes are most important, it is necessary to include them in discussions of end-of-life care. Families often wish to spare the patient what they perceive will be a painful discussion, but most dying patients know exactly what they want. Impending death is usually harder on loved ones than on the patient. So long as dying patients are treated with love and dignity, they usually have few requests.

Watching someone you love die is painful. While death may be welcome to a suffering patient, families are usually afraid to let go. This can lead to a unique phenomenon called prolonged dying. Somehow, patients sense when their families are not prepared to let go and hang on until everyone is ready for them to die.

Many hospitals insist that patients have a living will. They feel that patients should know how much intervention they want and communicate it to someone with authority. By telling doctors ahead of time what the cancer patient's wishes are, they will be respected. This does not mean that treatment will stop, but it will allow avoidance of suffering from invasive therapies that will not prolong quality life.

Hospice is an option that should be considered. It is fairly easy to find an inpatient or home hospice in nearly every community. Based on a concept formed in France centuries ago, and developed in the UK by Dame Cicely Saunders, hospice allows a dignified death by providing comfort without aggressive medical intervention. While the issue of using addictive painkillers led many doctors to under treat dying patients, that is no longer the case. It is now standard to use whatever medications are needed to provide pain relief.

Before making a decision in favor of hospice care, it is necessary to know if the patient's goal is to die at home or in the hospital, and what is best for the family. Can the patient be kept at home, or is a medical facility necessary? Combinations of in-patient and home care are possible, too. Most oncologists are able to help assess the needs of dying patients and their families and make appropriate recommendations.

It is often said that the actual death of a cancer patient is a relief for both the patient and the family. While no death is truly welcome, a cancer patient's death can be made a profound and spiritual moment. By the time death arrives, the ravages of the disease often make the departure from suffering a blessing.

Preparations for a funeral or memorial services should be openly discussed with the patient before death. This is a good way to provide a sense of closure. I hope that my cancer never comes back, but I already know exactly what I want done if it does and I die from it. Knowing that my ashes will be sprinkled on the top of my favorite mountain gives me a sense of peace. I can visualize myself surrounded by gorgeous vistas, clear air and nature. Knowing this final request will be granted helps make the process of dying easier.

I strongly encourage patients and their families to have a private time to say goodbye. Sometimes patients bring up topics that have not been raised for a long time, as if they need to clear the air before they die. There is no need for pretense, and conversations with terminally ill patients can be extremely satisfying. Their illness gives them permission to be totally open and honest.

∼ 10 ∼

FAMILY TIES

Cancer is as much an ordeal for the family as for the patient. My husband and children were at Disney World when I called them to give them the news. They immediately packed up and headed home. My husband later told me that the drive was a nightmare. He kept thinking that I was going to die, and that he would be left alone with the children. It was almost too much for him to bear.

Eventually, he began to see my cancer as a problem to be attacked and solved. I saw it as a process to be experienced. I later discovered that this dichotomy is common and may be related to the way men and women think. Men like to tackle problems, while women like to talk with others who have been through the same experience. This can be the source of strife.

I found the best way to deal with my need was to meet my girlfriends regularly for coffee. This helped ease the burden on my husband, and it felt good to educate the other women about breast cancer and bring them up to date about my personal experiences.

Another issue that spouses of cancer patients face is the

sense that no one is paying attention to <u>them</u>. The patient receives a great deal of attention, and the spouse may feel left out. For the most part, I think it is a matter of survival. Placing emphasis on yourself as a patient is necessary to fight your disease. Later on, you can transfer that energy to others. If a spouse has to take a back seat to the patient, so be it.

Children are another story. I tried to maintain a normal routine at home. We ate dinner together just about every night and followed our usual bedtime routine. At first we debated whether or not to tell the children that I had cancer, and decided that truth was the best approach. I was afraid they would hear something in the community and then not trust us. We decided to keep it simple: We told them that I had a sickness called cancer, and that I would need an operation followed by chemotherapy and radiation treatments. We used a book written by a physician and cancer survivor to explain it, and soon they were prepared for me to become bald.

When my hair began falling out by the handful, I decided to have my head shaved. We did it in the driveway. But despite our preparations, the children were frightened, and we all began to cry. They told me I looked ugly, and that I would embarrass them. They begged me to wear a wig. By a stroke of luck, I asked them if they wanted to jump in the pool. Then I explained that I could not swim if I were wearing a wig. Within minutes we were all swimming and laughing. They wanted to touch my head and rub it. From that moment on, they never mentioned my baldness. I was still "Mom" to them.

The truth is that children are very perceptive. They are

able to handle a lot more than we expect. My then 2-year-old was asked by his preschool teacher how I was doing… "They cut her boobies off, put in water balloons and now they pulled her hair out," he answered matter-of-factly. While part of me is sad that my children were exposed to such a difficult situation, another part knows they were enriched by the experience and will be more sensitive adults. To this day, they will offer to rub my back, asking me if it hurts. Their nurturing touch feels better than just about anything else I could imagine.

While it is natural to be concerned about the children of cancer patients, the patient's parents are often forgotten, particularly when the patient is an adult. There are no words to express the fear and sadness on my parents' faces when I told them about my diagnosis. It is contrary to nature that a child might die before the parents. My mother and I were very close, but my illness has brought us closer. Now that I am stronger, I am not sure who enjoyed celebrating my parents' 50th wedding anniversary, my parents or me. The party was a big milestone celebration, for all of us.

11

THE THREE "FS" OF SURVIVAL

Having discussed the value of family in the life of a cancer patient, I would like to add two other "Fs" that are equally important: friendships and faith.

Family is expected to come together in times of hardship, and mine did. What overwhelmed me was the incredible outpouring of love and support from my friends. Notes and cards full of caring and concern arrived by the dozen. One friend took my children every Monday afternoon so I could rest. Another friend arranged for months of delicious dinners to be delivered every other night. At first I was hesitant to accept these dinners, but I came to view them as ways of nurturing and sustaining my family. After I recovered and was able to make dinners for other sick friends, I realized that it feels as good to be the donor as the recipient.

When friends did not call, I felt somewhat estranged from them. I came to understand they were usually afraid of bothering me. Some would call my mother or husband to check on me for the same reason. Their thoughtfulness left me with many hours to practice introspection and plan my future life.

When I was first diagnosed with cancer, I blamed myself. Then I came to realize that bad luck and, possibly, genetics were involved. I had always struggled with the concept of God. Doctors are scientists, and I had difficulty reconciling God with my personal understanding about how the world evolved. Lying in my bed, too weak to get up, I had lots of time to think about my faith. I began to read books, articles and even poems for insight. Visualization tapes worked well for me, and I listened to one each day. At the suggestion of one of these tapes, I began to pray — not to a specific god or person, but just to pray. I prayed that I might be healed and be able to enjoy my husband and family for years to come.

One day as I lay in bed with these prayerful thoughts in mind, I felt a touch on my forehead. It was accompanied by a feeling of peace and an intuition that I was healed. From that day forward, I steadily improved. There were minor setbacks, but for the most part, I believe I will not die of my cancer.

Sometimes I think cancer was God's way of communicating with me. I had become lost in work and the accumulation of material things. I was constantly striving for more success. If my cancer had not stopped me in my tracks, I doubt I would have changed. My children would have been raised by nannies and would have had only a passing association with their mother. Whereas I had never thought twice about missing a preschool program, now I wouldn't miss one for all the world. While I used to feel that I was indispensable as a doctor, I know that there are other equally talented physicians to care for patients.

However, no one can take my place as a mother, wife, sister and daughter.

A trite saying really sums it up best: cancer has been very good to me.

12

Tips

Although I covered most of my feelings in the preceding chapters, the essence of living with cancer can be distilled down to a few tips:

• Remember that talking to someone with cancer is the same as talking to someone without cancer. From the patient's perspective, it feels terrible to be treated like a leper.

• Many people think they are being considerate by not disturbing the patient. However, patients often perceive that silence as rejection. Go ahead and call, write or email. Patients who are too sick to respond will not answer the phone or email back. I can assure you they will be grateful for the support, even if they cannot respond right away.

• Don't feel rejected if your efforts to visit and communicate are met with no response. There are days when patients do not have the energy for interaction. Trying to muster the strength to entertain friends can be daunting during therapy. If the patient wants you to be near, be content with just holding hands, listening to music or sitting quietly.

• Small deeds go a long way. A note, a small donation to a cancer organization...these are wonderful gifts. Don't send flowers... they die. Don't send candy...it is usually too sweet to eat.

• Humor is very important, especially in the face of a possibly fatal illness. I loved to hear jokes and often rented video comedies. Laughter is a great release and is proven to stimulate the immune system.

• Don't forget the patient's family. They may need more support and relief than the patient does. Offer to bring dinner, take the kids out for a meal or run an errand. Something as easy as picking up the dry cleaning can be a big help.

• Pray for the patient and their family. Many studies have shown that prayer is definitely beneficial in the healing process. To this day, I credit my health to a combination of excellent medical care and the outpouring of prayer on my behalf.

PART 2

SIX
LESSONS FOR
LIVING WITH CANCER

❦. Introduction .❧

Things have changed. When I was in seminary, we were instructed not to mention the word "cancer" in public, especially from the pulpit. The very word itself, we were told, would create fears and frustrations; people would resent it. While I suspected this was not good advice, I tended to go easy on saying the word "cancer" out loud. I was even known occasionally to advise a family *not* to tell the patient that cancer was there. I guess I hoped it would somehow go away. Some objected to my advice back then. Others ignored it. But most accepted it.

I know more now, and I offer my new reflections tenderly and timidly. Those with cancer and their families who have confided in me have been my teachers. Many others have helped me refine my thoughts. Dr. Melanie Bone, the co-author of this book, has expanded my horizons and helped me tremendously. She is a marvelous and caring doctor.

I have condensed everything I would like to share with you into six little lessons. You will notice the first letter of each lesson forms an acrostic of the word: C – A – N – C – E – R. These lessons are a result of the struggles I have had as pastor, and of the many friends and family members with whom I have shared the power and pressures of cancer, and the fears which begin the day the doctor says, "We think it is cancer, and here is what we think we should do next." I invite you to *A Journey Through Cancer*.

Richard M. Cromie, D.D.

— • —

❧ 1 ❧

CONQUER THE FEAR

One of the first things a person must do when cancer arrives is to **CONQUER THE FEAR**. Orville Kelly, the author of _Until Tomorrow Comes_, calls cancer the "phobia of our time." He says we talk about cancer as if it were a sinister force, an alien power with superhuman tendencies to annihilate its unsuspecting victims. Kelly's advice from three plus decades ago needs to be modified some, but it is basically still true.

Let us first look for a moment at what cancer is. In this disease, cells go wild and refuse to answer regulatory signals from the brain. Instead of living a normal life and dying as programmed, these "rebellious" cells multiply out of control. They spread throughout the body and threaten the health of the entire system. In fact, the origin of the word cancer comes from a word that means, "crab-like," named because it "claws" away at the other cells in the body.

Cancer is actually a group of diseases which fall into four large categories with several subdivisions in each. An increasing number of cancers can now be successfully treated. Thanks to researchers all around the world, we are winning the battle on several different fronts. It will not be long until we reach the hilltop and conquer the whole disease. Pray to God for guidance to continue.

There are basically six types of treatment. I applaud them all. I think the worst advice you can ever take is, "Don't let them fool and fiddle with you. They will ruin the remaining time you have left." I have heard this in many different disguises. Whether it is surgery, radiation, chemotherapy, hormone therapy, immunotherapy or bone marrow transplantation which is best for the individual patient, progress has become the hallmark of our time.

In my opinion, you owe it to yourself, your family and your future to allow those who with great devotion and brilliant minds research and treat cancer, to share the results and rewards with you and yours. I thank God for the concern, caring and skill of those who treat and cure cancer. In the forty-plus years I have worked with cancer patients, I have seen miracles from God and "miracles" from all these treatments. Many who are reading these words, and who stand in the background of this writing, are living witnesses. In more recent years, we have come to expect the treatments to work, and a cure to follow. They do so with increasing frequency.

A seventh treatment I want to mention is the healing power of prayer and the positive force of your faith. It has been especially valuable in my work. While it is quintessential to those of us who believe and practice it, prayer has never been known to hurt anyone. I have found that most people with cancer, no matter how much or how lit-

52

tle they say they believe, are pleased to know that others pray for them. The Bible says that the prayer of a righteous man (or woman) has great power in its effects, and it does. But any well-intentioned prayer will do. If you do not have experience to formulate your own prayers, read some out of a book.

I encourage you to help others be more open about the phobias they have regarding this disease. We communicate better as time goes on. Yet, I often find that couples, children, friends and families are reticent to speak about it. When it is over, I too often hear someone say, "We wasted so much time when we could have talked." Don't wait: do it now!

Calling a fear by its name can usually disarm it, and it loses its salient power. Then you can proceed to handle whatever comes with a rational, spiritual, and dynamic approach, and eventually overcome the fear. Making friends with your fears is worthwhile work. The first thing we need to do is to conquer the fear of the word. Presently cancer can be controlled. In many cases it can be permanently arrested. It often is cured. Our prayer is that one day soon cancer will be a disease of the past. Conquer The Fear!

— • —

~❧ 2 ❧~

ANTICIPATE A STRUGGLE

It will not be easy, but while you work on conquering your fear, you must also **ANTICIPATE A STRUGGLE**. Those who have been through cancer will tell you what a struggle it is. Dr. Bone mentioned it first hand in her writing. In his book, _In The Beginning_, author Rabbi Chaim Potok says, "All beginnings are hard, and especially those you make by yourself." Each of us can easily recall the first day of important journeys through unchartered seas: the first day in school, the day you lost your job, the day your boyfriend left you for another, the day of your divorce, the day your mother or father died, the long road home after burying a child. Those lessons were difficult, often devasting. With cancer you can add another. You must now surrender to frightening treatments, tests and more tests, an uncertain future, etc, etc, etc. Oh dear.

An old friend once likened the beginning days of cancer to the uncertainty of entering a tunnel that is long and dark, as if traffic had stopped inside the Lincoln Tunnel underneath the Hudson River with all the lights out. One day when we were driving through the long long tunnel of

Mount Blanc, between France and Italy, traffic did stop, for what seemed an eternity. My wife still trembles when we recall that episode. There is nowhere to go and nothing to do but wait, worry and hope for some eventual movement and a light at the end of the tunnel. It takes a tremendous amount of trust and concentration.

With cancer, struggles within the body, mind, soul, and emotions are real and often overwhelming. Another friend with cancer said, "I feel there is an alien in my body with the power to destroy me." Regrets, anger and depression are common. Whoever said, "Cancer is the loneliest disease in all the world," was right. There are some identifiable stages on the road to acceptance, but they are not as predictable as some people expect. It is a start-and-stop journey which you must walk by yourself. Nobody else can walk it for you. Whether it is the radiation room, the operating room, an MRI or CT scan, this is strange new territory to conquer. The way is often rugged and steep, but you can manage it. Believe it.

Sometimes the more difficult battle is looking in the mirror and seeing yourself as others see you. You will notice physical changes that will continue to take place. Watching your body age is hard enough, but when the time frame is condensed, it becomes an impossible chore. Some things help— like a good sense of humor, good friends or a new hat (as my mother used to say)—but never underestimate the battle. I had a dear friend who while in the hospital for treatment and whose hair had fallen out, put on a different hat each day. But she also made each visitor wear one of her hats while they were in the room. Everybody laughed. It will take all the energy you can muster. God bless you.

~~.3.~~

NEVER GIVE UP!

Thirdly, I advise you: **NEVER GIVE UP!** I have seen remarkable things happen in many corners of my ministry. I have watched people's lives open up to the future. I have often seen children in trouble take on new depth and meaning. I have watched marriages restored where there had been little hope. I have watched new dynamics redirect a family after death. When the Bible says that God can work all things together for good, I tell you it is true. Never give up!

When Winston Churchill was asked to deliver the commencement address at his old preparatory school at the age of eighty-plus, he gave the greatest graduation speech of all time. When the graduates had received their diplomas and the long, dreary recitation of speeches had ended, Sir Winston was introduced. He stood at the microphone, cleared his voice, leaned forward and said, "Never give up!" He backed away from the microphone, cleared his voice again, and barked again to the students, "Never give up!!" He looked around, cleared his throat a third time, leaned into the microphone and declared, "In conclusion, I want to tell you again, never give up!!!"

This advice can be applied in other areas of our lives. If you have a difficult child, never give up on that child! If you have a shaky marriage, never give up on the marriage! If you have an illness of the body, mind or soul, never give up! Your life has a purpose. It will continue to have meaning. The appearance of cancer does not change that.

For many years, I was very close to a wonderful woman named Ginny. She had cancer that entire time. She was a little "on in years" when it started. She could have settled in and acquiesced. No one would have blamed her. But she looked deep into her soul and psyche and somehow tolerated an endless stream of operations, radiation treatments and chemotherapy because, she said, "The good Lord above is not finished with me yet. I have more things to do before He is through with me."

I visited her each week for years. We shared the Sacrament of Holy Communion together. We prayed together. She asked me an endless number of deep, theological questions. She focused on the future, even simple events such as what Scripture we would read together the following week. Near the end of her journey, I asked her how she found the courage to fight on and on. She smiled at me and said, "Richard, I read your book. You told us, 'Never Give Up!'"

• • • • •

NEVER GIVE UP!

When things go wrong, as they sometimes will,
When the road you're trudging seems all uphill,
When the funds are low and the debts are high,
And you want to smile, but you have to sigh,
When care is pressing you down a bit,
Rest, if you must-but don't you quit!

Life is queer with its twists and turns,
As everyone of us sometimes learns,
And many a failure turns about
When he might have won had he stuck it out;
Don't give up, though the pace seems slow,
You might succeed with another blow.

Success is failure turned inside out-
The silver tint of the clouds of doubt-
And you never can tell how close you are,
It may be near when it seems afar;
So stick to the fight when you're hardest hit-
It's when things seem worst that you must not quit.

ANONYMOUS

A footnote is necessary here. One woman told me she thought it was permissible to give up when peace comes within, and all else is in order. At that time, you are ready to surrender to the One Who Gave You Life. She asked me to read Psalm 139 to her, and she surrendered within the hour.

O Lord, thou hast searched me and known me!
Thou knowest when I sit down and when I rise up;
Thou discernest my thoughts from afar.
Thou searchest out my path and my lying down,
    and art acquainted with all my ways.
Even before a word is on my tongue,
    lo, O Lord, thou knowest it altogether.
Thou dost beset me behind and before,
    and layest thy hand upon me.
Such knowledge is too wonderful for me;
    it is high, I cannot attain it.
Whither shall I go from thy Spirit?
Or whither shall I flee from thy presence?
If I ascend to heaven, thou art there!
If I make my bed in She'ol,
If I take the wings of the morning
    and dwell at the utmost parts of the sea,
    even there thy hand shall lead me
    and thy right hand shall hold me.
If I say, "Let only darkness cover me,
    and the light around me be night",
    even the darkness is not dark to thee,
    the night is as bright as the day,
    for darkness is as light with thee.

PSALM139:1-12
(Revised Standard Version)

$$\text{~4.~}$$

CALL FOR HELP

When it gets difficult not to give up, it is time to **CALL FOR HELP.** You do not need to be a lonesome hero or heroine. That was O.K. for John Wayne but not for you and me. The Bible says clearly that it is not good for man (or woman) to be alone. One of the biggest problems with cancer, especially when it endures for years, is that you must keep the struggle going by yourself. No one else can take your treatments for you. No one else can listen to your inner dialogue at three a.m. No one else can read your charts to you. However, people are there who can help you.

I trust God, as I hope you do. I adore the story of the man who, upon slipping over the edge of a huge cliff, caught onto a sturdy little tree mysteriously rooted about ten feet from the top of the cliff. Trembling and shaking, he cried out, "Help me! Help! Is there anybody up there to help me?"

"Yes," came a deep, calm, reassuring voice. "I am here. Trust me. Let go of the tree and I will take care of you."

Pausing for another terrified moment, the man shouted, "Who are you?"

"I am God," the voice responded. "Let go and I will rescue you."

After another brief pause, the man called back up: "Is there anybody else up there?"

So say we all. We trust God, but. . . . (as I said, a sense of humor helps, too!)

When Jesus had to face the pressures that his life thrust upon him, he cried out for help. He asked his disciples to watch with him in the Garden of Eden. When he needed more strength, he called them and asked them to help. When everything seems to have changed (although nothing has really changed, because *you* are still you), you can be sure there will be times when you will feel very much alone. Reach out for help.

I tell patients and their families that foolish pride should never stand in the way. Ask for help when you need it. Your physicians will help you. Hospice programs are available to provide good professional advice and care. The American Cancer Society can be a tremendous asset. Support groups everywhere can help. So can pastors, priests and rabbis. If you realize that friends and family love you, they can help too. No one can possibly know what you need unless you tell them.

• • • • •

To the friends and family of someone with cancer, I advise you to let the patient set the pace. Your needs as a loved one are important, too. You are worried and in another kind of pain. No doubt you have heard about the stages that patients go through. Well, they do and they don't. As I mentioned, I have never seen one stage depart completely before another arrives. Resentment and rejection never really go away, even when they yield a little to other feelings. Full acceptance almost never comes.

So, be there to help if the patient needs you or needs to talk. I often hear friends and family say, "I would have gone to see him, but I didn't want to bother him." I always think of saying, "Who is kidding whom?" Most people are afraid to go because they do not know what to say. That is normal. But it is better to go than not to go. You cannot do much, but at least you can be there. For the patient, loneliness can be as bad as the disease itself.

A friend of someone with cancer told me, "If I had only known how serious it was, I would have gone to see her." Well now, stop and think about that. We know how swiftly our time passes on earth. We have boundless testimony of the wondrous and worrisome ways in which the days move on, "like a weaver's shuttle, so do my days go by," says the Book of Job.

We know that life is fragile. Every one of us is a single heartbeat away from saying good-bye. There is almost never a "wrong word" to say. Usually no words are necessary, just an, "I'm sorry," and, "I'm here," is all you need to say. A smile, a card, a story or a borrowed prayer is sufficient for the day. Take a small gift with you, or a Bible verse or a poem.

Or deliver this book. Having read it yourself, offer to talk it over if the patient agrees. Dozens of times, I have been told by families that magic communication takes place when the patient and the family member or friend read and talk about _How To Live With Cancer_ (now _A Journey Through Cancer_).

Some family members have said to me, "I wish we could have talked, but he never seemed to want to." Perhaps he did not. We will never know. Perhaps he was protecting you, or thought he was. Keeping fear and pain from others often is the course a patient chooses, especially when he is the strong one, the household "provider."

But sometimes, the visitor is grateful not to have to bring the subject up and refuses to intrude. "Intrude, my foot," my father told me in the nursing home. While he did not have cancer, he said "I have been dying to talk to someone. Will you talk to me now?" One son told me he had to bring the illness up three dozen times. Finally his father opened up and talked. "It was wonderful. For the first time in our lives we communicated," the son said. I suggest you begin talking about frivolous things like a football game or the weather. Then progress to more serious things before easing in to the whole topic of how the patient feels. A joke can help shoo the goblins away.

I often envy doctors. They carry a stethoscope. It gives them something to do with their hands, something to hold on to. In the room where cancer lives, visitors usually go in empty handed, except for heart in hand. But when all else is said and done, it is better to be there and to share what love means, even when you do not know what to say, than not to be there at all. Cancer is lonely. Actions speak louder than words. We all need to be loved. Say it again: we usually do not receive help, unless we ask for it.

⌐ • ⌐

~e. 5 .~

ENJOY THE LIFE YOU HAVE LEFT

ENJOY THE LIFE YOU HAVE LEFT!   In many cases, the time left we are talking about turns into years and more years. The initial shock often seems to threaten that. But ten years from now, the world will be talking about decades of recovery time for all cancers, not months or years.

Sometimes though, it all caves in. What was a quiet stream turns into a raging flood in the narrow valleys of your soul. If you are not careful, it will engulf you. The best way to approach this crisis is to see it as a new mirror in which to see yourself. There is a time for everything under the sun. Live your life one day at a time.

Even God cannot make a life that is not fragile. A friend told me, "Once you think you are going to die, nothing else ever matters as much again." Think about the most significant things that have ever happened to you. Most of them are special little periods of time. The years and decades often blend together as one.

Epictetus was an old philosopher. "He used to pour out great and mighty thoughts about all sorts of stoical things around 100 or so A.D. in ancient Greece.

"We should take life as it comes," he said, "not demand what we desire!" Then he added, "A wise Providence governs everything, so even the calamities are part of a providential plan. Only fools are upset by things they cannot change or control." Good teachings!

Then one day he was stricken himself. In order to save his life, they had to amputate his leg. Now it was time to see the stuff Epictetus was made of. Preaching is one thing, losing a leg is another. This is what he wrote:

"I shall not divorce myself from the goodness of the universe because of a miserable little leg! I shall continue to believe that God is still in charge."

Amen, Epictetus! That's the way I'd like to say it. Why ruin everything because of a miserable little leg, or a miserable little pain, or a miserable little anything? God is still in his heaven. You are still on earth. Christ will see you through.

John Cowper Powys is one of my favorite authors. When he was qualified by age, he wrote a book called, _The Art of Growing Older._ I recommend it to you, especially if you are in your middle or later years. To paraphrase Powys, he wrote: "It is like a journey home after a long walk on the beach. I love it so much down along the shore. But, the closer I get to home, the more open my eyes become, and the more I look forward to the moment when I can sit down to rest from it all and to think through everything my walk has given me. I concentrate my vision on those rare occasions when I realize how precious is the remaining portion of my journey.

But I look forward to the time when I can lay it all down, go home and rest away through the long night."

The source of the problem is that we think we own our lives. We assume we have a right to 80, 90 or 99 years of unending joy. We believe the universe owes us happiness and peace for as many tranquil days as we choose to have. The Bible reminds us to number our days. "The days of our years are three score and ten, or even if by reason of strength, they be four score, they are full of sorrow and we soon fly away." (Psalm 90) You still do not know what any day will bring forth.

When the actor Harold Russell lost both of his hands, he wondered how he could ever go out to greet the world again. He said he finally realized: "It is not what you have lost that matters; it is what you have left." Be determined to enjoy each moment, day, and decade of your remaining life. Otherwise you will squander your most precious possession in the world— your time, and your time together with those you love. Not only cancer patients are guilty. We all can be guilty of squandering time. Emerson said, "It is only as time, with relentless fingers, snatches away the pages of our lives, that we realize how few and precious are the remaining ones."

There is no right or proper way to handle the shock or grief of learning to deal with cancer any more than there is just one way to handle the death of one you loved too much to lose. But the suggested course normally runs towards the positive. It is not what you have lost, but what you have left that matters. If you sit and feel sorry for yourself, or grouse and grumble until the end of time, it is your privilege to do so. But you and the others who love you will miss the most treasured times of all.

— • —

～ 6 ～

RENEW YOUR FAITH

The final step I advise you to take is to **RENEW YOUR FAITH**. I do not say it because I am a clergyman. I am a clergyman because I have to say it. People of all faiths testify that just when they have had enough, when they cannot stand it one moment longer, power from beyond comes to take them by the hand. Whatever your particular faith may be, God will comfort you so that you can comfort others. "We were utterly crushed, but that was to make us rely upon God and not on ourselves. He has delivered me, and I have placed my hope in Him that He will deliver me again," says the Scriptures.

Thomas à Kempis was a Roman Catholic scholar of the Fifteenth Century who lived a gentle, meditative life in Germany. When he was faced with lingering illness, he wrote: "I cried out to God, 'Oh Lord, how will I ever make it to the end?'

Then, I heard a little voice whispering back to me: 'Thomas?'

'Yes.'

'Did I ever fail you? When you were a little child, did I not carry you in my arms? When you faced the passions of your youth, did I not deliver you from all their might? In the reigning view you had over the top of your middle years, and when you walked too near the fire, have I ever failed you, Thomas?'"

Thomas said meekly, "No, my Lord, no, you did not!"

The voice said, "Well what makes you think that I would fail you now?"

"I have been young and now am old. Yet I have not seen the righteous forsaken, nor his children begging for bread!" (Psalm 73)

Thomas à Kempis responded, "No, no, you have delivered me and you will deliver me."

The Bible adds, as we have said, "I have placed my hope in Him that He will deliver me again." And aye, He will. You cannot live without a renewal of your faith. Whatever that means to you in the little world where you live and dream, I encourage you to renew your faith.

Orville Kelly is a man in whom cancer was discovered many years ago. Rather than be defeated, he became the founder of **Make Today Count**, a helpful organization where people with cancer have gathered for many years to talk about what they can do to help themselves, each other, their families and to the world. There are many ways to help if you want to, or where you can receive help if you are ready to receive it. Kelly wrote the following prayer:

> *Give me the strength to face each night before the dawn*
> *Let me count each passing moment*
> *As I once marked the fleeting days and nights,*
> *And give me hope for each tomorrow.*
> *Let my dreams be dreams of the future.*
> *But when life on earth is over*

Let there be no sadness –
Only joy for the golden days I've had.
AMEN.

"Only joy for the golden days I've had." Annie Dillard wrote in her prize-winning book, *Pilgrim At Tinker's Creek*, after her young brother-in-law died. "The dying always say 'Thank you,'" she wrote. "They never say please."

Thank you Lord, for life, for all that is good and for all that death can never touch.

⌐ • ⌐

POEM FOR THE LIVING

When I am dead,
Cry for me a little.
Think of me sometimes,
But not too much.
It is not good for you
Or your wife or your
Husband or your children
To allow your thoughts to dwell
Too long on the dead.
Think of me now and again
As I was in life,
At some moment which
It is pleasant to recall.
But, not for long.
Leave me in peace,
And I shall leave
You, too, in peace.
While you live,
Let your thoughts
Be with the living.

ANCIENT INDIAN PRAYER

MELANIE BONE, M.D.

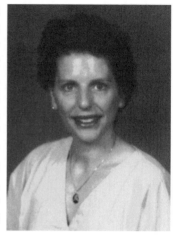

Dr. Melanie Kaye Bone was born in upstate New York in 1960. She was raised in Albany until she went away to high school at the Phillips Exeter Academy in New Hampshire. Dr. Bone studied Russian language and English Literature at Georgetown University before returning to Albany for medical school. She did her internship and residency at George Washington University Hospital in Washington, DC. She moved to Florida to enter into private practice in 1991.

For the first 9 years in Florida, Dr. Bone practiced with a large group and then left in 1999 to open her own solo office. Just one year later she was diagnosed with breast cancer and stopped working for almost a year to finish her treatments. She now works part time in an office close to her home.

Dr. Bone is married to Bill Bone, a trial lawyer. They have four children – Becky 8, Carlton 7, Bailey Mae 5 and Rex 4. In her "spare time" she participates in many community-related activities. She is President of the Hope Project, a mobile mammogram unit that provides free and low-cost mammograms to underserved women in Palm Beach County. Dr. Bone serves as Treasurer of the Florida Obstetrics and Gynecology Society which represents over 1,000 obstetricians and gynecologists across the state of Florida. She is on the Board of the Florida Breast Cancer Coalition, a grass roots advocacy group and is also active in the Young Survival Coalition, an international organization devoted to the needs of women under the age of 40 with breast cancer.

As a result of her cancer experiences, Dr. Bone started a not-for-profit company called ChemoComforts, Inc. ChemoComforts produces kits to help get through cancer treatments. The website, www.chemocomforts.com provides more information about this endeavor.

74

RICHARD M. CROMIE, D.D., PH.D.

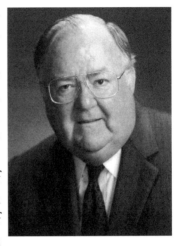

Dr. Richard M. Cromie has been the Preaching Pastor at the Royal Poinciana Chapel in Palm Beach, Florida, since 1995. The Chapel is a historic non-denominational church founded by Henry Flagler. The original building is over 100 years old.

Dr. Cromie is a native of Pittsburgh, Pennsylvania. He is a graduate of both the University of Pittsburgh and the Pittsburgh Theological Seminary, with honors. He received his Doctor of Philosophy degree from St. Mary's College of the University of St. Andrews in Scotland. He also has a Doctor of Divinity degree from Grove City College. He and his wife Peggy have three daughters: Catherine DeCramer of Charlotte, North Carolina; Anne Campbell Pentolino of Gainesville, Florida; and The Rev. Courtney Beth Cromie of Boca Raton, Florida. They also have two grandchildren, Maddie and Wil.

Dr. Cromie served several Presbyterian parishes in the Pittsburgh area before his 1983 departure to be Senior Pastor of The First Presbyterian Church of Fort Lauderdale. He is co-author of *The Future Is Now,* author of *Sometime Before The Dawn, How To Live With Cancer, Christ Will See You Through, You Now Have Custody Of You, The Rhapsody of Scripture, and When You Lose Someone You Love,* all available from Desert Ministries, Inc.

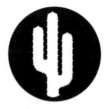

DESERT MINISTRIES INCORPORATED

Desert Ministries is a non-profit corporation devoted to the development of helpful materials for use by those in special need. It provides books and booklets for clergy and for laity on a variety of subjects. Information on other publications will be sent upon request. A sample packet will be sent without charge if you ask.

Recent publications include: *When You Lose Someone You Love, How to Help an Alcoholic, Christ Will See You Through, God's Promises and My Needs, You Now Have Custody of You, When Alzheimer's Strikes, When a Child Dies,* and more.

Desert Ministries, Inc.
P.O. Box 788
Palm Beach, FL 33480

wwww.desmin.org